ALL ABOUT
ASTHMA
AND ITS
TREATMENT
WITHOUT DRUGS

ALL ABOUT
ASTHMA
AND ITS
TREATMENT
WITHOUT DRUGS

By David Potterton ND, MRN, MNIMH
Consultant Medical Herbalist and
Registered Naturopath

foulsham

LONDON • NEW YORK • TORONTO • SYDNEY

foulsham

The Publishing House

Bennetts Close, Cippenham, Berkshire, SL1 5AP

ISBN 0-572-02153-4

Copyright © 1995 W. Foulsham & Co. Ltd.

Phototypeset in Great Britain by Typesetting Solutions, Slough, Berks
Printed in Great Britain by St. Edmundsbury Press, Bury St Edmunds.

Contents

Preface

Asthma is a serious condition, which can be treated by herbal and naturopathic methods.

This book is an introduction to these methods and how they can help people who have been properly diagnosed as suffering from asthma or a closely related respiratory disease. It shows that there are alternative options available to lifelong treatment with drugs.

Many of the natural remedies mentioned are available from herbalists or health food shops, while others may be obtained only after a consultation with a registered medical herbalist or naturopath.

It is strongly recommended, however, that where doubts about treatment arise it is advisable to seek the personal advice and encouragement of a qualified practitioner. This book is not intended as a replacement for proper medical diagnosis and care, and should not be regarded as such, but it should, I hope, be a doorway to the world of complementary medicine which is now so rapidly being universally accepted.

Note: Because it is recognised that there are contra-indications and that individuals may react differently to herbal remedies, the author and publishers emphasise that they cannot be held liable for any adverse effects caused by self-treatment with any of the remedies mentioned in this book. Self-treatment must be undertaken according to the individual's own judgement.

The Natural Treatment of Asthma

A severe acute attack of asthma is a fearful experience – the victim never knows whether it will gradually pass and normal breathing will be restored, or whether it will become worse with tragic consequences.

Although the statistics have been questioned, it does seem that not only are more people suffering from asthma, but that a higher number of people are now dying from it than ever before.

Why should this be so when physicians have never had so many sophisticated drugs at their disposal?

Is it because we live in an age where the leading medical philosophy has concentrated the approach of doctors on choosing a chemical palliative?

"I'm afraid you have asthma Mr C, just take these drugs and you should feel very much better. Use this inhaler in the morning, this one in the afternoon and this one before you go to bed. You don't want to wake up in the middle of the night gasping for breath do you?"

Relatively little interest is expressed in the patient's lifestyle – how much exercise he gets, what he eats, or even how he breathes.

Contrast this with a herbalist's or naturopath's approach. The practitioner is interested in the patient as a whole – he needs to know not just *that* the patient has asthma, but *why* he has it.

This means delving into the patient's general level of health, lifestyle and family background, for that is where the answer will be.

Is there a history of wheezing, respiratory infections, or allergy? Is there a postural problem, or emotional distress?

Is the diet wholesome? Does the patient breathe correctly? Does he get enough exercise? Is the patient's work a contributory factor?

No stone should be left unturned in arriving at a rational basis for treatment – a treatment that will be tailored to each individual case.

It will almost certainly mean a change to a healthier lifestyle. It may involve eliminating certain foods from the diet and adding in others. It may be necessary to take nutritional supplements and herbal or homoeopathic medicines for a while to treat the underlying aspects of the disease.

Giving someone with asthma a pharmaceutical drug that merely dilates the lungs, may deal with the presenting symptom, but it seems inappropriate when given con- tinuously, perhaps for several years. It may, as some medical reports have suggested, even worsen the condition in the long term.

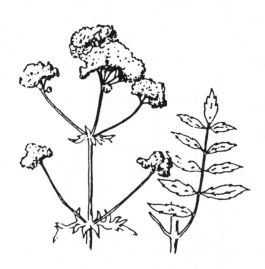

Valerian

Words of Caution

Herbal medicines are generally safe, but they are not without contraindications. Therefore, the following general rules should be observed:

1 Never take any herbal medication during pregnancy without advice from a qualified practitioner.

2 Do not treat babies and young children, or the very elderly, without obtaining professional advice as dosages are much more critical.

3 Do not take herbal medicines without advice if you are also taking medicines from your own doctor, as the two may interact.

4 Do not self treat if you are suffering from a liver condition, heart problem, or other serious disease.

5 Always use herbs and herbal products from reputable herbal medicine suppliers, but preferably from a medical herbalist.

6 Do not gather medicinal herbs from the wild. Do not use other than culinary herbs from your garden.

7 Self-medication should be undertaken only for short periods of time and for simple conditions. Do not self-treat undiagnosed conditions.

Chapter 1

The Growing Asthma Toll

About two million people in Britain suffer from asthma and nearly 2,000 die from it every year, despite claims by the medical profession and pharmaceutical companies that there have been amazing advances in understanding the disease.

Of those who die from asthma – and there is one death every four hours – four in every 10 are aged under 65. This is a tragic waste of life.

The cost of orthodox treatment now exceeds £400 million a year, with 20 per cent of this being spent on the 100,000 people who are admitted to hospital as emergencies.

These costs do not include the more than seven million working days lost each year due to asthma sufferers being forced to take time off.

Why is this disease getting out of hand?

One suggestion has been that because the condition is now better understood, more people are being correctly diagnosed and treated. But if this was so one would expect the death rate to be drastically reduced.

Another suggestion, backed up by clinical evidence, is that it is the overuse of bronchodilator drugs that may be the cause of the trouble.

Doctors in New Zealand, concerned at the death toll from asthma in their country, investigated whether continuous use of inhalers could be detrimental rather than beneficial to their asthma patients.

About 90 patients with mild to moderate asthma took part in an experiment – they were to use their bronchodilators continously for five months and then use them only when they felt they needed them for a further five months. However, a placebo – a powder similar to the drug to be inhaled was substituted for the real drug half of the time.

The patients were allowed to continue to use other prescribed asthma drugs, such as steroids, when required.

The results showed that most of the patients had better control over their asthma when they did not use their bronchodilators on a regular basis, but that they were also better when they were inhaling the placebo, rather than the real drug.

In addition, most of those who also took steroid drugs for their asthma, were better during the placebo phase of the study.

The doctors reported* that, although regular bronchodilator treatment was recommended by asthma specialists as a method of reducing the severity and frequency of asthma attacks, it actually had an adverse effect, causing the patient's control of the disease to deteriorate.

These findings support the observations of naturopaths over many years that simply giving a drug in complete disregard of the patient's lifestyle deals only with the symptoms and not with the disease.

Thus the result is that the disease is likely to get progressively worse and out of control so that, according to the logic of asthma specialists, even stronger drugs become necessary.

More than 70 years ago naturopaths were taught that with drug treatment asthma patients would continue wheezing miserably to a good age when they would die from the effects of the drugs they were taking.

Now, it seems, a substantial number cannot even expect to live to a good age.

If we go back further, to the turn of the century, we find that the standard medical school teaching was that asthma was never a cause of death. How times have changed.

I appreciate that it may be difficult for asthma sufferers, particularly those on strong medication, to believe that their condition can be ameliorated by natural methods, but my experience is that most cases of asthma will respond to simple herbal remedies and naturopathic treatments as outlined in this book.

The Lancet, 1990, 336, 1391

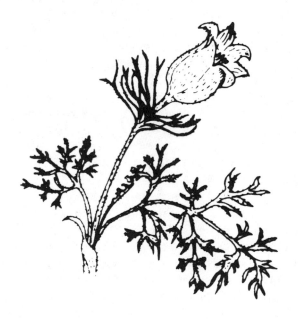

Pulsatilla

Chapter 2

What is Asthma?

The word "asthma" comes from the Greek language and means gasping for breath. The disease was known to Hippocrates, the father of medicine, more than 2,000 years ago, but was first clearly described by the Greek physician Aretaeus sometime between 200 and 300 AD.

The chief symptom of asthma is the severe wheezing, or "dyspnoea" which tends to occur in isolated attacks. In between the attacks, the sufferer appears to be quite free of the disease.

During an attack, the bronchial tubes, particularly the smaller ones become narrowed, either because of a build up of mucus or because of an acute reaction to a specific food or allergen which causes the tubes to go into a spasm. There is usually an inflammatory process also taking place, causing the tubes to swell.

As the attack subsides the tubes relax and return to their normal diameter and breathing becomes easier again. Mucus may be coughed up.

Asthma affects children as well as adults and the total symptom picture may vary from one individual to another, but there are two main types – those whose wheezing is due to a specific allergy, such as food colours or dust mite and those whose wheezing is triggered by food and drug intolerances and common irritants, such as smoke, fumes and dust. Emotional factors may exacerbate the attacks. Often there is an overlap between the two types.

Naturopaths and medical herbalists are not just concerned with the triggering agents which cause the wheezing, but also with the background factors which determine the underlying state of the lung cells, such as family traits, diet, posture, breathing, exercise and environmental pollutants.

The importance of such factors has been confirmed by the observations of surgeons who transplanted lungs from donors with asthma into recipients who had previously never suffered asthma. The transplanted lungs, instead of becoming healthy, continued to be asthmatic. The reverse was observed when lungs from asthma-free donors were transplanted into asthma sufferers: the lungs remained free of asthma.

This means that the underlying tissue state of the lung is the important factor, because this is what *predisposes* an individual to the disease. The triggering factors are responsible only for the acute symptoms. Orthodox medicine concentrates on treating the triggering factors. Herbalists and naturopaths also treat the predisposing factors.

CHILDREN

Asthma is the commonest chronic disease in children with twice as many boys as girls affected by it. Are we to blame heredity for this? Not entirely – and particularly when a disease affects an estimated 10 per cent of the childhood population: nature just does not make such large statistical errors.

It may be true that one or both of the parents also suffered asthma, or hay fever, or a related disease like eczema, but this does not imply that the disease is automatically handed down. It is not.

What may be handed down is a specific tissue type which predisposes an individual to the disease but, more frequently, it is a family's eating habits and lifestyle that are "inherited". Also important are the parents' nutritional state, both deficiencies and excesses, prior to conception and the mother's nutritional state in pregnancy.

In brief, the disease is an interaction between an individual's tissue state and lifestyle, or life circumstances.

The tragedy is that as many as 45 children a year die from asthma in England and Wales alone. They often have a history of coughing at night, repeated lung infections, including bronchitis, ear infections, tonsillitis and bouts of wheezing after exercise.

There are dietary considerations in all of these conditions and, therefore, they need to be treated properly and not just with antibiotics or inhalers.

When an acute asthma attack develops, the constriction in the bronchial tubes due to spasm and plugs of mucus makes breathing extremely difficult with exhalation more difficult than inhalation. This leads to over-inflation of the lung cells and a build up of carbon dioxide in the blood vessels. If there is a concomitant lung infection the outcome can be grave.

ADULTS

In adults asthma affects more women than men and tends to be more severe with chronic wheezing. Allergy as a triggering factor is said to be not so common. The picture resembles chronic bronchitis with attacks of coughing and production of sputum.

The attacks often accompany colds and flu, or are triggered by irritants, such as dust, perfumes, paints, tobacco smoke, emotional upsets and exercise.

Chapter 3

Importance of Accurate Diagnosis

As there are a number of conditions related to asthma – and a few unrelated ones – which also produce wheezing it is important that a correct diagnosis is made. For example, the most common cause of wheezing other than asthma is congestive heart failure. This would obviously occur in an elderly rather than a young patient, but it is not uncommon for an elderly person to suffer both asthma and heart failure.

With asthma there is usually a previous history of hay fever, rhinitis or bronchial catarrh. Eczema, urticaria, or tummy upsets after eating certain foods may also be complained of by the sufferer, or they may occur in close relatives.

Other causes of wheezing in older people include renal asthma, due to poor kidney function, and lung cancer.

Status asthmaticus is a particularly severe form of asthma in which the wheezing may continue for several days and which usually requires hospital admission.

Emotional stress is also common in asthma and is an aggravating factor.

During an acute attack the patient finds exhalation difficult and, therefore, the chest becomes expanded. The breathing is noisy and the condition makes it difficult to talk except in gasping sentences.

Skin testing for sensitivity to animal and plant proteins may reveal a specific allergy. Blood tests can also give important information.

Lung tests are useful to monitor the progress of the disease and to warn of a decline in lung function. They are carried out with a spirometer into which the patient breathes out as hard and as fast as possible. A measurement can be made of both the volume of air and the speed at which it is exhaled. When the lung is operating normally about seventy-five per cent of the air is exhaled within one second. In asthmatics the time increases depending on the severity of the lung spasm.

Analysis of sputum by a laboratory when asthma is due to allergy can reveal the presence of cells known as eosinophils. In blood tests these cells are found to be be increased in allergic conditions.

One of the simplest investigations, however, is with the use of the stethoscope. In asthma the practitioner will hear a magnification of the continuous wheezing noises called rhonchi, which contrast with the bubbling and clicking noises heard, for example, in bronchiectasis.

X-rays are mainly required to rule out the presence of a foreign body or tumour in the lung.

Naturopaths and herbalists may perform some or all of these investigations, or may refer the patient to a centre which has the necessary equipment.

Chapter 4

Related Respiratory Conditions

A number of respiratory diseases, some serious, cause breathing difficulties which, to the untrained, resemble the wheezing in asthma.

HAY ASTHMA or HAY FEVER

Many people are sensitive to grass, tree and summer flower pollens, which make them wheeze, sneeze and suffer with streaming eyes and noses throughout the spring and summer.

Affected individuals are said to suffer from a type one, or atopic allergy. The wheezing is due to constriction of the lungs following a series of events involving the production of antibodies and their attachment to specific cells which are abundant in the lungs and respiratory tract.

These cells contain histamine which is released when the pollen enters the respiratory tract. The effect of excessive histamine circulating in the blood is over-production of mucus, swelling of mucous membranes and blood vessels, and contraction of muscular tissue in the lungs. All these events create wheezing and the hay fever symptoms. The orthodox medical approach is to prescribe anti-histamines in an attempt to quell the symptoms.

The naturopathic and herbal approach is to deal with the tissue state which makes the individual sensitive to pollens. Postural and breathing exercises are important. Some of the herbal medicines described later in this book are helpful in this condition. Homoeopathic medicines, such as Mixed Pollen, can be used rather like vaccines to desensitise the system. See the chapter on homoeopathy and follow my recommendations on diet.

EMPHYSEMA

A serious lung disease which can develop in people who have previously suffered severe asthma attacks, but frequently occurs in those who suffer chronic bronchitis. It most often appears in those aged over 60. The constant breathlessness in emphysema is due to a loss of elasticity in the smallest bronchial tubes as a result of enlargement and damage to the vessel walls.

The disease is common in those who smoke or who have been exposed to inhalation of dust. A mild form, due to ageing, occurs in many elderly people who have never suffered a respiratory condition.

Early treatment for emphysema is essential otherwise only palliative measures can be given. A number of herbs described in this book are helpful.

BRONCHIECTASIS

This disease affects all age groups and is due to enlargement of the bronchial tubes, following a respiratory infection associated with bronchial obstruction: for example, whooping cough, or the entry of a foreign body into the lung. There is usually an abundance of mucus and breathlessness. Herbal medicines can be helpful.

BRONCHITIS

A serious disease which causes a significant number of deaths each year in the winter months. It is commonly associated with smoking, or inhalation of irritating chemicals, which damage the lung, setting up an inflammatory process and predisposing the lung to infection. There is production of sputum and, consequently, breathlessness and a chronic cough.

Unless properly treated, the condition becomes worse each winter and complications, such as emphysema and heart failure may follow. Early and appropriate treatment is essential. A combination of orthodox and herbal medicines together with naturopathic techniques may be necessary. The sooner an individual embarks on natural treatments the better.

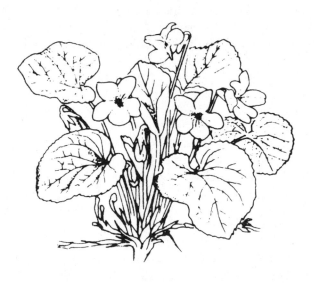

Chapter 5

Drug Induced Asthma

Aspirin and other anti-inflammatory drugs, particulary those used in the treatment of arthritis, can cause asthma in susceptible people. This is a pity because aspirin is a versatile drug which has found a new indication in recent years as a preventive treatment for stroke.

I can sympathise with those who are "allergic" to aspirin as I, too, am sensitive to this drug and have never been able to use it. It can cause intense wheezing in those who react to it and is potentially fatal.

Fortunately, herbal medicine can offer alternative treatments for arthritis and for aspirin's other indications.

Although aspirin is now made synthetically, it was originally manufactured from salicin, an active principle of willow bark *(Salix alba)*. The use of willow in treating pain and fever was described by Hippocrates, and used by herbalists down the centuries, but discarded by physicians until the 19th century.

Although salicin containing herbs, in addition to willow bark, are commonly prescribed by herbalists, their therapeutic indications vary somewhat from those of synthetic aspirin.

The "allergenic" profile of the herbs may also vary so that people who do react to aspirin may not react to the herbs. As far as I am aware there has been no research undertaken by herbalists on this fascinating subject.

However, it is well known that attacks of wheezing in some people are induced by citrus fruits, particularly oranges. Interestingly, oranges contain a substance similar to acetyl salicylic acid from which aspirin tablets are made.

Another related substance is tartrazine, the yellow dye, which is still used by a few food and confectionery manufacturers despite all the adverse publicity that it has received as a cause of asthma and allergies.

Tartrazine was also used extensively by drug manufacturers, including those producing asthma drugs, to colour their tablets yellow. The pharmaceutical industry has now discontinued the use of this agent.

A survey revealed that of 149 bronchodilator drugs, 29 contained tartrazine, while a further 59 contained other colouring additives. Obviously people whose asthma was triggered by tartrazine would find that their asthma drugs were making their asthma worse.

One can only remark that this is yet another historical example of so-called scientific medicine being not very scientific, and certainly far from natural in its approach to disease. Another example is the use of a solvent in the manufacture of aminophylline, a drug used to reduce bronchospasm. The solvent has been found to cause asthma in susceptible individuals.

Note: People with arthritis who are taking anti-inflammatory drugs from their doctor and who find that they are suffering bouts of wheezing are advised to consider herbal and naturopathic treatments for their condition.

Chapter 6

Earlier Days

If we go back to the 1850s we find that well known and successful herbalists, such as George Slack of Derby, had quite a good understanding of asthma. In his *Treatise on the Pathology of Disease* he classified asthma under two headings: moist asthma accompanied by a discharge of heavy mucus; and dry, nervous or spasmodic asthma with no expectoration. Today we would call those bronchial asthma and allergic, or atopic, asthma.

The causes of the disease were said to include breathing in the fumes of metals and minerals, being in a foggy atmosphere, or breathing in impure air, exposure to draughts, impaired digestion and violent exercise.

HERBAL RECIPE

Among his recommendations was to make up a cough powder from 1½oz each of powdered Liquorice root, Marshmallow root, and Anise seed, 4oz of Elecampane root, and two small teaspoonfuls of powdered Cayenne.

Half an ounce of this powder was then combined with half an ounce each of Yarrow and Horehound.

Two pints of boiling water were poured over the mixture which was reduced in a hot oven to 1½ pints. It was then strained and bottled. The dose was a wineglassful up to six times a day.

Chapter 7

Posture and Breathing

I have never yet met anyone with asthma who has been told anything about posture or correct breathing by their family doctors. Neither have I met anyone – at least not in recent years – who has had their chest measurements taken – and yet these, one must assume, have an important bearing on respiratory disease.

Doctors are all too eager, it seems, to restrict their services to prescribing inhalers.

More attention, in my view, should be paid to correct posture and breathing. The person who has poor posture is usually a poor breather. They may also have a negative mental attitude to life.

It can, of course, operate the other way round: negative feelings in early life may be the predisposing cause of poor posture and a contributing factor towards asthma.

It's as if the individual lacks confidence in himself and wants to hide away by shortening his height – a form of symbolic cringing – instead of presenting a bold appearance.

SUFFOCATED

I have met people with asthma who complain that they have felt suffocated all their lives, because their parents would not let them express their feelings, or because they

25

were afraid at school. They are not necessarily aware of the association between these experiences and their disease. But during a consultation the association emerges and the awareness is developed.

There can be no doubt that many diseases, including asthma, can have psychosomatic threads to them – they are the manifestation of interactions between mind and body. Unhappy early experiences can leave their mark in this way. Obviously, this is more easily diagnosed in some people than others, but the wise practitioner should always search for it in his asthma patients.

There are other possible reasons for poor posture – the school desk and satchel, for example. It has been observed that most children enter school with perfect posture and leave it with their postures damaged due to spending 16 years or more at desks and in seats that are inappropriately designed. They also struggle home with bulging satchels on their backs which throws the spine out of alignment at a critical phase of development.

Naturopaths are very aware of the effects of poor posture and breathing on the metabolic processes of the body. But I was also pleased to meet, many years ago, a consultant orthopaedic surgeon at the Royal London Homoeopathic Hospital, who was very enthusiastic about good posture.

He was of the view that the posture we develop in early life, whether good or bad, usually remains unchanged for the rest of our lives. He went as far as to claim that good posture could delay the degenerative processes of the ageing body. He was particularly aware of the serious effects that bad posture had on the severity of arthritis, and he noticed that people who continuously adopted a slumped posture developed various diseases.

He also equated a person's posture with their mental attitude. He tended to think that good posture was the result of a positive attitude.

Fortunately, it is not too late for anyone to improve their posture, and consequently their asthma. Postural re-education has always been an important part of naturopathic medicine, although in recent years there has been a growing sub-group of complementary therapists, who describe themselves as teachers of the Alexander technique.

They specialise in teaching the postural philosophy and techniques of Mr F. Matthias Alexander, who wrote several books on this and related subjects in the early part of this century.

An improved posture certainly aids the respiratory function, while better breathing improves liver function. On inhalation the lungs press into the liver with a massaging effect which helps the body's detoxification processes, including the eradication of allergens. The build-up of waste products and irritants in the blood and in the lungs, perhaps over many months or years, is an important factor in the development of respiratory disease.

This is an example of how the body's organs are interdependent and not – as some would have us believe – a collection of components which are best treated chemically.

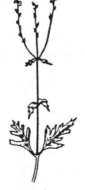

Vervain

Chapter 8

Fasting – A Potent Treatment

Fasting under the supervision of a naturopath is one of the most potent treatments for asthma. An attack of wheezing can be stopped within a few hours. Indeed, it should be a rule that no food should be taken during an asthma attack, provided there are no other contraindicated medical reasons.

I appreciate that this is rather different from the practice of allowing the patient to eat what they like provided they use an inhaler three times a day. But the latter philosophy will never cure the patient. Properly directed fasting, however, can given long-lasting results, even in long-standing cases.

During a fast the sensitivity of the respiratory organs to allergens diminishes rapidly. Any inflammation present in the lungs is quelled, and any respiratory infection is dealt with more efficiently.

In severe, longstanding cases of asthma, better results are achieved by entering a residential naturopathic clinic which specialises in fasting. In such an environment the attitude to fasting is more positive and it can be undertaken for longer periods of time. There are no concerned relatives, putting you off with intimidating questions such as: "Do you really think you are doing the right thing going without food?"

Many people find that they feel better for fasting at home

on one day a week, or by modified fasting for three or four days.

A short, strict fast is not the same as starvation. One is allowed – at the discretion of the naturopath – soups and broths, plus pure unsweetened fruit and vegetable juices and herb teas. For short-term fasting at home one is allowed to eat fruit and some salad items, plus soups and broths, and to drink fruit juices and herb teas.

What is restricted is everything else – red meat, poultry, fish, dairy products, cereals, including bread, and drinks such as tea, coffee, alcohol and squashes.

It is important to make sure the bowels are emptied prior to fasting. This is usually helped by a day on fruit only and, if necessary, by a dose of a herbal aperient.

Although specialist clinics may recommend fasting for two to three weeks for some conditions, I have never found that necessary for asthma. A modified fast for up to a week is usually long enough for a beneficial result.

I would recommend any reader who is contemplating a fast to first read a more specialist book on the subject and to consult a naturopath about the best way to proceed.

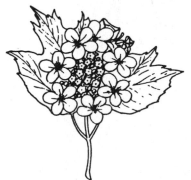

Cramp Bark

Chapter 9

Cleaning Up – with Fruit and Vegetable Juices

Fruit juices are widely available, but it is debatable whether they are entirely a natural food. Early man would have lived off the fruits of the forest, but in most cases he would have eaten the whole fruit rather than just the juice, thus providing himself with the important fibrous part as well.

The same applies to vegetables. It is more natural to eat a carrot than it is to drink carrot juice, but the drinking of carrot and other vegetable juices has, in recent years, become equated with healthy living, possibly because of the advent of mechanical juicers for domestic use. Previously, the juice had to be pressed out.

Of course, it is just as unnatural to boil vegetables and then throw away the water, because a lot of goodness is literally being thrown down the drain.

I contend that for health, food should be eaten as whole as possible and as unprocessed as possible, on a regular daily basis. This means that fruit is best taken whole rather than just extracting the juice. If the juice is taken it should be diluted and not taken concentrated.

However, the use of fruit and fruit juices for medicinal purposes has long been part of naturopathic medicine. It is not unusual for a patient to be recommended to take only fruit or dilute fruit juices for a day or two as part of a cleansing process, or to restore an alkaline balance to the system.

Normally, it is better to drink diluted fruit juices to quench one's thirst rather than drink tea, coffee or alcohol, and it is better to eat the whole fruit rather than consume too much juice.

But it has to be remembered that some forms of asthma are commonly aggravated by fruit, particularly citrus fruits. And not everyone seems naturally able to digest fruit adequately – about one in six people, for example, are unable to digest oranges.

However, in the treatment of asthma a number of fruit and vegetable juices have been found to be of benefit in a good proportion of cases and, consequently, have found their way into naturopathic medicine.

Carrot juice is just one of the more popular. It is a rich source of beta carotene, from which the body produces vitamin A and it is anti-microbial – it thus helps to prevent infections of the respiratory tract. The beta carotene has also been shown to have anti-tumour properties.

I do not agree with those practitioners who think that one should drink it until the skin turns yellow. This, say the enthusiasts, is a sign that the carrot juice is doing its job. On the contrary, I would say that it is a sign of over-dosing. Also, excessive amounts of vitamin A are toxic to the liver.

An advantage of carrot juice is that it forms a good base into which other juices can be mixed. Spinach, which is also rich in vitamin A, is a natural partner of carrot in the treatment of asthma, but because its taste is rather stronger, it is best combined in the ratio of one part spinach to two parts carrot. Spinach juice is, of course, a well known source of iron.

Celery juice, which can be given in equal parts with

31

carrot juice, has a reputation as an anti-arthritic treatment, but it is also useful in asthma, because of its mineral content.

Like spinach it is rich in iron. So, too, are parsley juice, apricot juice and raisin juice. You may wonder how you get juice out of a raisin. The method is to wash the raisins and then soak them overnight in enough water to cover them. The raisins, which have absorbed some of the water, are then put through a juice extractor and the rest of the water added to them. Grape juice can be added to taste.

Parsley juice is another rich source of vitamin A. It is a very potent cleanser of the blood and of the kidneys and, therefore, smallish doses only are taken. It can be combined with carrot juice in the ratio of one part parsley to seven parts carrot, but on its own one should not take more than a tablespoonful as a single dose.

Grapefruit juice, is a popular drink, rich in vitamin C and also contains a respectable amount of vitamin A. It can be recommended in asthma if there is no allergy to it.

For home use, I would advise a wineglassful of the juices or combinations as detailed above two or three times a day.

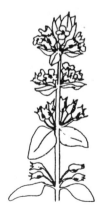

Thyme

Chapter 10

The Role of Herbal Medicines

Plants were accurately described and classified by herbalists and botanists long before physicians decided to do the same with common diseases.

It was Thomas Sydenham who decreed in the 1600s that physicians should reduce diseases "to certain determinate kinds with the same exactness as we see it done by botanic writers in their treatises of plants" – a decree that lasted well into the 20th century.

There is merit on both sides, of course. It is just as important to be able to identify plants accurately and to know which ones have the best properties for treating asthma and other lung conditions as it is to be able to distinguish accurately between various respiratory diseases.

The individual characteristics of herbal medicines for asthma and other respiratory conditions have been well described throughout history, and modern research into plant constituents has confirmed time and again the validity of the observations of the early practitioners.

Among herbal medicines indicated in asthma are those which are antispasmodic and which help to relax the bronchial tubes; the expectorants which unclog the lungs by increasing the ability to cough up foul mucus; circulatory stimulants which boost blood flow away from the congested lung; and demulcents which soothe irritated lung tissue.

Pollen from non-poisonous plants which are known to trigger the acute symptoms of hay fever and wheezing can be used in small doses throughout the season to build resistance.

For example, elderflowers, which can cause wheezing, sneezing and watery eyes in susceptible people when in full bloom, can treat the condition when a fluid medicine made from the fresh flowers including the pollen is taken in doses of a few drops every day.

This is similar to the homoeopathic principle of like curing like, although the medicine is not a homoeopathic one. This method is used by a number of practitioners including myself.

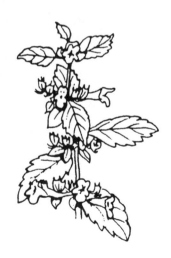

Lemon Balm

Chapter 11

The Lung Strengthener

There are several varieties of thyme, but the Common Thyme *(Thymus vulgaris)* is considered to be the most valuable for the respiratory tract, possibly because of its reputation in calming the paroxysms associated with whooping cough.

Its antispasmodic properties are useful in asthma and its antiseptic action, largely due to its content of thymol, a volatile oil, make it a front-line remedy in bronchitis.

Although it is cultivated as a culinary herb, the thyme that grows wild in its natural habitat in southern Europe is more robust and yields higher amounts of the volatile oil.

Another variety known as Mother of Thyme, or Wild Thyme *(Thymus serpyllum),* which grows all over Europe, has similar indications, but is not so potent in action and does not have such a marked aroma as Common Thyme.

According to Nicholas Culpeper, Common Thyme "purges the body of phlegm", which would seem to support its use in bronchial coughs, chesty catarrh and bronchitis, and is "an excellent remedy for shortness of breath". Culpeper also described Thyme as a strengthener of the lungs.

The volatile oil in Thyme is related to turpentine, the oil distilled from pine wood, which traditionally has been used as an inhalation in bronchitis to soothe the respiratory tubes.

As a herb, Thyme can be used as a tea, or made into a syrup and given in tablespoonful doses. For an infusion use about one teaspoonful to a cup of boiling water, sweetened with honey. Strain the mixture before use. A syrup is made with a double-strength infusion to which honey or raw cane sugar rich in molasses is added in the ratio of about 1lb of sugar to one pint of infusion.

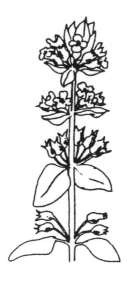

Thyme

Chapter 12

The Cough Stopper

Coltsfoot is one of the most popular cough remedies – even its botanical name *Tussilago farfara* gives a clue as to its use. "Tuss" means cough, which is why cough medicines are described as anti-tussives.

People with asthma will find Coltsfoot soothes the bronchial tubes and also helps to get rid of excessive mucus on the chest. It is commonly used in combination with Horehound and Marshmallow.

The plant grows on waste ground, but is also found on the banks of rivers and in wet places. It is a little unusual in that the flowers precede the appearance of the leaves. Medicines are made from the flower stalks as early as February, from the flowers in March and April and from the leaves, which are shaped like horses' hooves (hence Coltsfoot) in May, June and July. The plant is a rich source of mucilage.

Herbal cigarettes are not as widely available as they once were, but smoking dried Coltsfoot leaves was a popular treatment for respiratory complaints.

A decoction is made by placing an ounce of the leaves in a quart of water and simmering until one pint is left. The mixture is then strained and honey added. It is taken in wineglassful doses two or three times a day. A syrup, made from the flower stalks, is indicated in bronchitis, the dosage being one or two teaspoonfuls three or four times a day. Fluid extracts and tinctures are available from medical herbalists.

Chapter 13

The Mucus Reducer

One of the most popular lung tonics with a long history of use, White Horehound is an expectorant which has the interesting property of reducing excessive bronchial secretions.

It is of use, therefore, in catarrhal affections and bronchial asthma in which there is abundant mucus. Traditionally, it was included in mixtures for bronchitis, coughs and colds and few households were without it.

Known to herbalists as *Marrubium vulgare,* it is a bushy, perennial plant with woody stems, growing to about two feet high. It is found throughout Europe, and can withstand, even prefers, dry poor soils, flourishing at the roadside and on waste ground. It has a white flower which is produced in midsummer.

As an expectorant for coughs it is usually combined with other pectoral tonics, such as Liquorice, Coltsfoot and Marshmallow.

A syrup can be made by adding honey to a double strenth infusion. A *standard* infusion is made by pouring a pint of boiling water on to one ounce of the dried herb and allowing to stand until cool. It is then strained and taken in doses of two fluid ounces.

A hot infusion induces sweating and is a useful standby in mild fevers as it helps to reduce the temperature. Where there is lung involvement the same treatment will help relieve congestion.

Horehound has one or two other properties which have to be taken into consideration by those prescribing it. These include its ability to promote the menstrual flow and its laxative effect in large doses.

BLACK HOREHOUND

The Black Horehound *(Marrubium nigra* or *Ballota nigra)* has similar properties, but is more popular with some practitioners. Its antispasmodic properties are useful in coughs and asthma. It is best taken in the form of a tincture or fluid extract and in combination with other pectoral remedies rather than an infusion because it has a bitter, unpleasant taste.

Like the white, it also has an effect on the female hormone system helping to regulate the menstrual cycle and, in addition, is relaxing to the heart and circulation and may lower blood pressure.

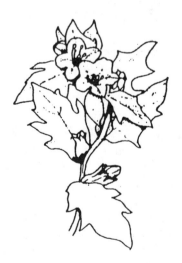

Horehound

Chapter 14

The Lung Relaxer

Respiratory medicines made from Lobelia have a long history of use. Galen, the most distinguished physician in the Roman empire, gave his stamp of approval to it in the second century AD and it has retained a place in pharmacopoeias until modern times.

Lobelia is one of the more important remedies used by medical herbalists as it is considered to be a potent relaxant. However, it is also an expectorant, a diaphoretic and a respiratory stimulant, which makes it a valuable remedy in bronchial asthma.

Lobelia was very popular with American Indians who used to smoke it in their "peace pipes". Some of the alkaloids present in the plant resemble nicotine and it has been used as a substitute tobacco to help addicts give up smoking.

It was also one of the plants traditionally used in inhalation therapy for asthma and bronchitis. The leaves would be combined with those from other very potent plants like Stramonium and burned in the sick room. The patient would inhale the fumes to obtain relief. This was certainly safer than taking potent plant remedies internally.

In less than large doses Lobelia induces vomiting and was used for this purpose by one 19th century school of medicine as a means of clearing the stomach and respiratory passages of putrid matter. As far as I am concerned this form of "emetic therapy" with Lobelia, belongs to the age of routine purgings and bleedings and is no longer taught.

I do not know of any professional herbalist who uses Lobelia to induce vomiting to clear accumulated mucus from the respiratory passages, although this indication has been published in popular herbals in recent times. Should emesis be necessary, as in the case of poisoning, there are better remedies available.

In the long history of conflict between herbal practitioners and physicians in the United States, Lobelia was itself dubbed a poison, presumably because it can induce vomiting. In one famous case a physician accused a herbalist of poisoning his patients with Lobelia and the herbalist was brought to trial. The outcome, however, was that the herbalist was acquitted.

A professor at Yale gave supporting evidence that he had used Lobelia for 27 years in large amounts and for long courses of treatment without experiencing any ill effects.

There is no doubt that Lobelia has been used to save countless lives, but that because of its emetic properties and great potency it must be used with the utmost caution.

Modern herbal students are taught to treat Lobelia with respect and to use it in specific ways – in a syrup or vinegar, for example, or as a plaster or poultice in the treatment of swollen joints.

For bronchitis and asthma, it must be used in herbal mixtures in correct proportions and rarely on its own. It is combined with other expectorants, relaxants, or stimulants according to the individual case. *This remedy must be taken only under supervision of a medical herbalist.*

Chapter 15

The Chinese Spasm and Allergy Remedy

How long does it take Western orthodox medicine to realise the usefulness of a herbal treatment? Well, in the case of one particular Chinese herb, Ma-huang, it took about 5,000 years.

This herb, known botanically as *Ephedra sinica,* is the source of the alkaloid, ephedrine, which has been used by doctors since the 1920s, either on its own or in combination with other compounds, to treat bronchial spasm and allergic respiratory conditions.

However, the ephedrine that is sold by pharmaceutical companies is not the natural ephedrine, but a chemical copy of it, which can be manufactured in the laboratory.

Unfortunately, the use of ephedrine in isolation, can give rise to unpleasant side effects. While it relaxes the bronchial muscles, which is a useful property, it also raises blood pressure.

Large doses may give rise to a number of symptoms, including muscular weakness, trembling and anxiety, nausea and vomiting, headaches, sweating, insomnia and palpitations.

It cannot be given, therefore, to people with high blood pressure or coronary heart disease and is contraindicated in those with thyroid disease or with prostate problems.

Ephedrine has similar effects on the body as adrenaline, a hormone produced by the adrenal glands. We produce adrenaline in response to stress and, therefore, giving ephedrine in the dosage needed to stop an asthma attack can make the sufferer feel as if they are suffering a panic attack – the heart beats faster, the pupils dilate, the lungs take in more oxygen and the skin turns pale.

These effects are due to stimulation of the sympathetic nervous system, and drugs and other agents which produce these effects are known as sympathomimetics. Indeed, in earlier times, adrenaline was given by injection as an asthma remedy.

It often happens in a severe acute attack of asthma that the fear it produces causes the body to release enough adrenaline to abort the attack.

Although it is an effective bronchodilator, ephedrine has become less popular for this purpose due to its side effects. However, at lower dosages ephedrine is still used as a preventive treatment for asthma, and there is some evidence that the natural ephedrine from the plant causes fewer side effects than the synthetic version.

Medical herbalists, in preparing their medicine from the plant, do not isolate ephedrine but extract *all* the plant's properties, including ephedrine, from the stems. This makes ephedra a much safer remedy. For example, although ephedrine in isolation causes an increase in blood pressure, this has not been recorded as an effect of the herb.

Even then, it is usually prescribed in combination with other remedies that act on the respiratory system. It is also indicated in emphysema and hay fever.

Ephedra is an important remedy in herbal medicine but, because correct dosage is important and because it is not suitable for everyone, it is recommended that it be taken only under the supervision of a properly qualified herbalist.

Chapter 16

Dealing with Bronchial Catarrh

The California gum plant, a shrub with yellow flowers, provides an anti-asthmatic medicine, which until 1949, was listed as an official drug in the British Pharmacopoeia.

It has been used by herbalists as an ingredient of their medicines where asthma accompanies bronchial catarrh, because the plant, otherwise known as Grindelia *(Grindelia camporum),* is also an expectorant and loosens mucus trapped in the lungs.

It has also been used as a whooping cough remedy to ease the frightening whoops or paroxysms. In medical circles the fluid extracts of Grindelia and Liquorice were combined and added to a mucilage.

Its use by herbalists, however, goes back hundreds of years. It is, for example, one of eighty expectorants listed in the Indian Materia Medica.

Like many plant remedies it has additional properties and, in the case of Grindelia, it also acts on the kidneys and bladder as a diuretic.

Also like many plant remedies, dosage level is important. While it has been used for kidney and bladder affections, such as cystitis and catarrhal discharge, it is not suitable for prolonged use or in liberal amounts. Correct dosage activates the kidneys: overuse irritates the urinary tract.

In herbal medicine, Grindelia is usually combined with

other expectorants or asthma remedies, according to the individual case. Using remedies in combination increases the therapeutic action required and reduces unwanted side effects.

A traditional combination is one part Grindelia, mixed with one part each of Thyme, Horehound and Coltsfoot. One ounce of the mixture is steeped in one pint of boiling water. Then add 5ml of tincture of ginger, or a teaspoonful of powdered ginger, and 1ml of peppermint essence. Sweeten with honey if necessary. A dessertspoonful can be taken three times a day.

As a single remedy Grindelia should be taken only under the direction of a medical herbalist.

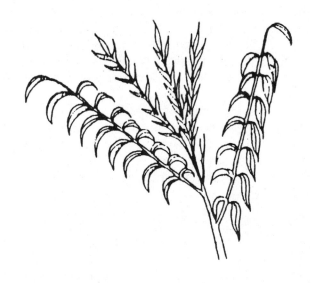

Liquorice

Chapter 17

The Asthma Weed

When a plant is known to country folk as asthma weed, there is obviously a good reason for it. This is the name given by people in Queensland, Australia, to *Euphorbia pilulifera,* a member of the spurge family.

A tincture made from the plant, which thrives in tropical climates, was once listed as an official medicine in the *British Pharmacopoeia,* as were other compound remedies containing the plant's active principles. It was used not only for asthma, but also for bronchial coughs and inflammatory lung diseases. It is still found on the dispensary shelves of medical herbalists and is still among herbs recommended as anti-asthmatic in some "health books" and herbals.

The problem with Euphorbia, as far as domestic use is concerned, is that it comes from a large family of plants, many of which are poisonous, and could be easily confused with other remedies. For example Euphorbium, a related plant, is a drastic purgative which has fallen into disuse.

There is no doubt, however, that Euphorbia is a useful asthma remedy, provided proper attention is paid to dosage. As only a few drops of the tincture constitutes a single dose I can only recommend that it be taken on prescription from a medical herbalist who will, no doubt, use it in combination with other respiratory medicines according to the symptoms involved.

Chapter 18

The Lungworts

Lungwort is the common name of two different plant remedies – *Sticta pulmonaria* and *Pulmonaria officinalis* – both of which are used in modern herbal practice for respiratory complaints, but which are not entirely identical in use.

While herbs are continually referred to and sold under their common names, it is important as a general rule that the correct botanical name is known, otherwise unfortunate mistakes can be made. These two remedies have led to confusion even among writers of herbal books.

Sticta pulmonaria is an asthma and hay fever remedy, which is anti-inflammatory and soothing. It is also useful in sinusitis, the common cold, influenza, coughs and catarrh. Combined with red clover flowers it has been used for whooping cough and croup.

This Lungwort is a moss which grows on oak and beech trees and is also known as Oak Lungs and Lung Moss.

Pulmonaria officinalis is a common garden plant, formerly found in woods and shady places, producing small purplish flowers and spotted leaves. It was the leaves which attracted herbalists in earlier times as, according to the Doctrine of Signatures, they seemed to resemble the shape of the lungs.

Surprisingly, the doctrine which states that a sign in the plant reveals what diseases it can be used for, held true –

the leaves, made into a medicine, certainly relieved various lung diseases. This Lungwort is soothing to irritated lung passages and is used in coughs, bronchitis, pharyngitis and bronchial catarrh. Culpeper recommended the plant "for coughs, wheezing and shortness of breath".

Lung syrups are made from both remedies, or they can be taken by infusion. Tinctures and fluid extracts are also prescribed by medical herbalists.

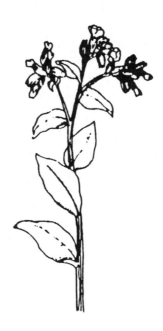

Lungwort

Chapter 19

Asthma and the Senega Indians

In the 1730s a Scottish physician who was living in Pennsylvania learned of the healing properties of a plant used by a tribe of American Indians for treating snake bites.

The plant was known as snakeroot. The doctor observed that the symptoms caused by the bite of the rattle-snake resembled pneumonia, so he experimented by using the plant as a medicine for a number of respiratory diseases and found that it was surprisingly effective. The remedy helped to loosen the chest of phlegm, increased the flow of urine and activated the sweat glands. He had to be careful with dosage, however, because the plant was also emetic. In overdose it causes severe vomiting and purging.

By the 1740s the medicine was being used in Europe for respiratory complaints and became known as Senega, after the Senega Indians.

The plant is still used by medical herbalists in mixtures for chest complaints, but it is contraindicated in pregnancy because it increases the menstrual flow.

Although traditionally an infusion of Senega was taken in small doses, in modern practice it is always combined with other lung remedies to obtain its positive effects and to reduce undesirable ones. I therefore recommend that Senega is not used at home as a single remedy, but is taken on prescription from a herbalist who will dispense it in a correctly balanced mixture.

Chapter 20

Pleurisy Root

An important remedy in modern herbal practice, Pleurisy Root was used by both Canadian and American Indians as a lung medicine to aid expectoration and to reduce inflammation and breathlessness.

It is particularly effective in pleurisy, helping to reduce pain, which is how it came to get its name.

Herbalists, however, know it as *Asclepius tuberosa* and find it useful in a wide range of chest diseases involving production of mucous which is difficult to cough up, or where it is necessary to reduce fever.

Because of its antispasmodic property, it is frequently incorporated in mixtures for asthma.

The root is harvested from a perennial plant which flourishes in North America and which grows to about half a metre, producing yellow-orange flowers in late summer. At one time it was an official remedy in the US pharmacopoeia.

In large doses Pleurisy Root is emetic and purgative and, therefore, care must be taken with it. I would not recommend it for home use unless it is being taken under the supervision of a medical herbalist.

It is best combined with other remedies. A popular combination is one part fluid extract of Pleurisy Root to two parts Composition Essence (obtainable from herbalists). The dosage is 5ml (a teaspoonful) in half a glass of hot water. Such a remedy improves circulation, helps to reduce temperature in colds and chills, and improves the elimination of morbid matter via other channels.

In feverish, flu-like diseases Pleurisy Root is added to mixtures which help to reduce temperature naturally by inducing sweating. Such a mixture might also include Yarrow, Horehound, Bayberry and Boneset, with small amounts of Capsicum and Ginger.

In coughs it is often combined with other expectorant remedies like Horehound, and in asthma with other antispasmodics like Wild Yam.

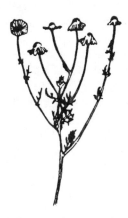

Chamomile

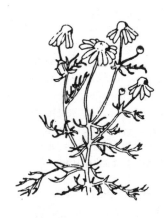

German Chamomile

Chapter 21

Homoeopathy for Asthma

Homoeopathic medicine is a branch of natural therapeutics and is widely employed by many naturopaths in the treatment of asthma.

The remedies are generally without side effects, although some people who are allergic to lactose may be unable to take homoeopathic tablets.

In my view the major task of homoeopathic medicine in asthma is to correct the underlying constitutional state of the patient.

But there are other important indications: for example, where an emotional state exacerbates asthma attacks.

The ability of homoeopathic remedies to act rather like vaccines which can be taken at the same time as the disease – unlike orthodox vaccines which are taken prior to the onset of a disease – underlines their usefulness in both acute and chronic asthma states.

Although they can be, and are, used to ameliorate severe acute attacks, their success often depends on the selection of the correct remedy in the individual patient.

The effect is not a blanket one, like the bronchodilatory effect of asthma drugs, it is, on the contrary, very individual. One needs to select in a specific dose the substance, or one similar, that is responsible in that individual for causing the bronchoconstriction.

It is obvious, therefore, that the disadvantage of

homoeopathy is that what will be an effective medicine in one person might be totally ineffective in another.

However, because the action is entirely different from an asthma drug, the homoeopathic remedy can be used alongside any drug treatment that the patient may have to resort to.

Of course, in the real world, most sufferers from asthma are usually taking strong-acting drugs to control their symptoms, and will know how effective these are in their own case.

They are then able to monitor quite well any added benefits they get from taking homoeopathic remedies and will be able to be weaned off their drugs as their underlying health improves.

Although many people are under the impression that herbal medicine and homoeopathy are similar, there is, in fact, a vast difference.

Herbal remedies are produced only from extracts from plants, while homoeopathic medicines are made from dilutions of a wide range of substances, including poisons. One remedy currently available, although not for asthma, is made from the arrow poison used by the bushmen in South Africa.

It can be worrying to a new patient to see that he has been prescribed "arsenic", when he has actually been given this substance in a dilution which is non-toxic, but at a dose designed to stimulate the body's immune system. Manufacturers might consider this possibly disturbing confusion in naming products.

Like other systems of medicine, homoeopathy has evolved and many practitioners now prescribe a cocktail of remedies to cover all the symptoms presented by the patient. This resembles the prescribing method of herbalists who generally give a mixture of remedies, in any given case.

Among the homoeopathic remedies that have been found useful for the underlying constitutional state in asthma subjects are:

ARSENICUM ALBUM

This is the white oxide of arsenic made into a solution and then potentised according to homoeopathic pharmacy methods. It is given to the anxious, restless patient, who tends to wake in the early hours with a wheezy cough.

BELLADONNA

The medicine is made from the fresh flowers of the deadly nightshade *(Atropa belladonna)*. It was introduced into medicine by the father of homoeopathy, Samuel Hahnemann, who used it as a treatment and vaccine for scarlet fever. It is also used for asthma and for bronchitis which comes on suddenly. In asthma it is indicated for those who cough and perspire a great deal.

BRYONIA

A tincture is made from the root of the white bryony and it is from this that the homoeopathic dilutions are manufactured.

This is the remedy for when a cold always goes to the chest. In asthma, the picture is one of irritated lungs with a dry cough. It can also calm those who suffer from extreme nervous irritability.

CARBO VEGETABILIS

This medicine, made from vegetable carbon, or charcoal,

usually from either the beech or birch tree, helps the patient who feels stifled and requires plenty of fresh air in the room.

They feel better if the air is kept circulating by a fan, or if a window is kept open, even in mid-winter. It can also relieve wind which builds up in the stomach causing breathlessness.

THUJA

Herbalists and homoeopaths both consider *Thuja occidentalis* to be a deep acting remedy. Known also as the Tree of Life or Yellow Cedar, Thuja is a coniferous tree found in North America.

The homoeopathic remedy is indicated for conditions like asthma and eczema when it is due to a previous vaccination. Often, the onset of asthma follows a vaccination in childhood, but the remedy has been used with success even when it is the child's mother who has been vaccinated.

This is not the place to become involved in a discussion of the merits or otherwise, of orthodox vaccinations, but it is obvious that when a vaccination is given, products associated with the disease against which protection is being sought, are being introduced into the bloodstream, and it is these, or other products used in the manufacturing process which act as a trigger in asthma.

YERBA SANTA

An evergreen shrub found in California which has been used in herbal medicine. The homoeopathic remedy helps to increase expectoration in asthma and bronchitis when the cough is dry.

VERATRUM ALBUM

The root of the White Hellebore, which grows in the alpine regions of central Europe, contains veratrine, a potent alkaloid. Its use in medicine has been restricted because of its poisonous nature.

However, as a homoeopathic medicine it has been found useful in asthmatic attacks accompanied by a cold sweat.

NATRUM SULPHURICUM

Some patients are worse in dry, hot climates, while others are affected more by damp foggy weather. For the latter constitution, a homoeopathic dilution of Nat. sulph. (sodium sulphate) is indicated.

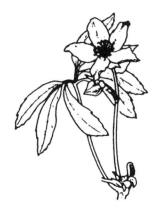

Black Hellebore

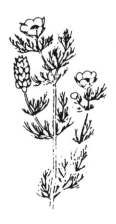

False Hellebore

Chapter 22

Diet and Asthma

People with asthma require a nutritious diet, free from artificial additives, as so many of these can cause attacks.

Although food manufacturers have been forced to reduce the number of additives in their products in recent years due to pressure from food conscious consumers, and some additives have been banned, a considerable number are still in use. Indeed, many processed foods cannot be produced safely without incorporating certain additives. However, people with asthma should reduce these foods to a minimum.

There is no doubt that a significant proportion of asthma cases are due to sensitivity to these foods. There are, for example, at least 30 food additives which have been reported to cause attacks of asthma.

They include food colours, food preservatives, anti-oxidants and flavour enhancers. I recommend that a specialist book, such as *"E For Additives"* by Maurice Hanssen, be consulted for details of adverse reactions caused by food additives.

I appreciate that it is very difficult in the modern world to live totally on additive-free food, particulary for those who have an active social life. If one is continually telling one's hosts: "I cannot eat that," then invitations tend to become less frequent, unless the hosts are very understanding.

Different countries still have different rules about permitted additives, so going on holiday can also have implications for asthma sufferers. But it is important to avoid processed foods as much as possible.

Some asthmatics are sensitive to everyday foods, such as milk, eggs, wheat, nuts, citrus fruits and fish. It is not clear whether the sensitivity is due to the basic food or to some chemical used in its production, such as antibiotics, pesticides and sprays or cleaning agents.

In these cases one may need the help of a practitioner in identifying the culprit food items and to make sure that elimination from the diet does not result in an unbalanced diet. However, it is quite simple to exclude these food items from the diet for a short period of time to see whether any improvement takes place.

In addition to these considerations it is advisable to follow a diet that does not weaken the body's immune system. Full resistance against disease can be gained by excluding all devitalised foods from the diet.

Foods that should be omitted are: white sugar, white flour, white rice, white pasta, and all products made from them, including white bread, refined cereals, biscuits and cakes; jams, confectionery, particularly chocolate, alcoholic beverages and excess amounts of tea and coffee. The consumption of red meat should also be reduced.

All foods that create mucus, such as cream and milk, should be omitted. Condiments, particularly salt which evidence now suggests aggravates asthma, are best avoided.

The intake of organically-grown vegetables should be dramatically increased together with fruits and fruit juices, unless there is a specific allergy to any fruit (see Chapter 9). Only whole grain cereals should be used.

All food should be chewed thoroughly to avoid indigestion, which in some people can induce wheezing.

The adoption of a good, wholesome diet as described here is an essential step on the road to recovery.

Chapter 23

Herbal Preparations

A number of herbs which are used in the treatment of asthma, such as Fennel, Elderflowers, Liquorice and Valerian, can be bought as herbal teas, or in powder or tablet form, from health stores and other retail outlets, but the advantage of consulting a medical herbalist is that an individually made up herbal medicine will be prescribed.

The herbalist may also dispense a mixture of herbs from which a "tea" can be made at home.

When the medicinal properties of a herb are soluble in water, infusions and decoctions are an acceptable way to take them.

Herbalists do not believe, however, that home-made or shop bought medicines should be taken on a long-term basis without proper supervision or for undiagnosed or serious conditions.

It is also inadvisable to take herbal medicines at the same time as taking drugs prescribed by a doctor without appropriate advice as there is the possibility of an interaction.

Although herbal medicines have been used safely for thousands of years, many modern chemical drugs are known to interact with foods and, consequently, may do so with herbs. This is not the fault of the herbs. Any interaction is a problem created by the introduction of drugs containing chemicals, the molecules of which are not and have never been present in nature. They have been created in a laboratory and are totally foreign to the natural world.

In making infusions and decoctions care must be taken not to exceed the dosage range of the more potent remedies.

INFUSIONS

Infusions, also known as teas or tisanes, are usually made with the softer parts of the plant, such as the flowers or leaves.

These are chopped finely and about an ounce placed in a jug, or teapot with a close fitting lid. A pint (20 fluid ounces) of boiling water is poured onto the herb and the lid is placed on.

The herb is infused for 10 to 15 minutes, stirring occasionally. When ready the tea is strained off. The usual dosage range is from half to two fluid ounces two or three times a day.

For domestic purposes one fluid ounce is approximately equal to to 30ml or two tablespoonfuls. (For those who prefer the metric system one ounce in weight is equal to 28 grams and a pint is equal to 568ml).

If the medicine is to be taken under supervision on a long-term basis half an ounce to one pint of water is usually recommended.

When a combination of herbs is being used to make an infusion the total amount still does not exceed one ounce per pint.

DECOCTIONS

Decoctions are more suitable for the harder parts of the plant, such as the bark, roots and berries. To every ounce of plant material, which is best ground down into a rough powder, or finely chopped, 1½ pints (30 fluid ounces) of cold water is poured on and the jug covered. This is then allowed to stand overnight.

The mixture is then brought to the boil and simmered for 20 minutes, or until there is a pint (20 fluid ounces) of liquid left.

The decoction is strained and given in doses of from half to two fluid ounces two or three times a day.

Infusions and decoctions can also be made in a coffee percolator.

TINCTURES

These are used when the medicinal properties are either destroyed by heat, or not sufficiently soluble in water.

The herb is steeped (macerated) in a mixture (known as the menstruum) of alcohol and cold water – usually a minimum of 20 per cent pure alcohol – for at least two weeks before being pressed out and filtered ready for use.

The tinctures prescribed by medical herbalists are usually made commercially with pure alcohol for which a government licence is necessary. They may also undergo the process of maceration and filtration several times in order to strengthen the tincture and to reduce the final alcohol content to a minimum.

Tinctures can be made with brandy, but this is a rather expensive process. However, the preparation is much stronger than a simple infusion or decoction, the ratio being 1:5 – one ounce of the herb to five fluid ounces of menstruum. Most tinctures need a 25 per cent proportion of alcohol to water. Dosage ranges from 10-40 drops (½ml-2ml), except for the more potent remedies. The advantage of tinctures is that they are more convenient to use and they keep well.

Some herbalists prefer tinctures made in the ratio of 1:3 – one ounce of herb to three fluid ounces of menstruum. On filtration the amount of tincture recovered is made equal to the original amount, that is three ounces, by making up the amount with further menstruum, or by re-maceration.

FLUID EXTRACTS

Strong tinctures, or fluid extracts, are made by reducing the final amount recovered. This is achieved by evaporation on a very low heat for several hours using a water bath, or double saucepan.

An official fluid extract is one that contains the equivalent of one ounce of herb to every fluid ounce of extract (a ratio of 1:1) and contains an adequate amount of alcohol to preserve it.

DOUCHES

Medicinal preparations such as lotions, mouth washes, gargles and douches can be made from infusions. They are filtered after straining off the herb.

INFUSED OILS

Herbs, such as Calendula and Comfrey are steeped in a bland oil, such as olive oil, in a warm place – traditionally in the sun – for at least two weeks so that the medicinal properties are infused into the oil. They are then strained ready for use.

Infused oils are excellent for external use and, therefore, the strength may vary. The infusion process can be repeated by adding more herb to the oil and setting aside for a further time.

In the treatment of asthma a practitioner would use a specific infused oil for massage and manipulation to the chest and back to improve circulation and to help remove irritating waste from the lungs.

ESSENTIAL OILS

These are oils extracted direct from the plant. Many are diluted and used mainly by aromatherapists for simple massage and beauty treatments, but medical essences, including peppermint, eucalyptus and cinnamon oil, for example, are prescribed in small quantities by herbalists for internal and external use.

As a number of essential oils are toxic, even when considerably diluted, *they should not be taken internally without expert knowledge.*

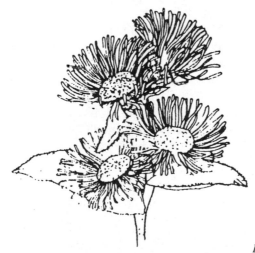

Elecampane

Chapter 24

A Herbal Selection

Herbal medicines have been used since the dawn of time to treat asthma and other lung diseases, including bronchial coughs and catarrh, bronchitis, emphysema and bronchiectasis – diseases in which the patient's ability to breathe has been mildly or seriously affected.

This section contains a description of botanic remedies frequently prescribed by herbalists to help alleviate these diseases.

It also includes remedies which have a more general toning effect on the whole body.

Herbalists and naturopaths always treat their patients as whole people rather than as a collection of components.

Do remember that caution with all medicines, including herbs, is advised during pregnancy. While most are safe, a few are contraindicated and, therefore, should be taken only under supervision of a qualified practitioner. The same caution applies to the treatment of babies and young children.

Agrimony

Agrimony
AGRIMONIA EUPATORIA

Also known as	Church Steeples
Where found	Throughout northern Europe
Appearance	A strong growing herb with green/grey leaves covered with soft hairs. Flowers are small and yellow on long slender spikes.
Part used	Herb
Therapeutic uses	A good general tonic for the whole system. It is a good liver cleansing remedy and will help to clear the skin of pimples, blotches and other eruptions. Culpeper recommended it "to cleanseth the breath and relieve the cough". The dried leaves taken as an infusion are useful in treating simple diarrhoea and general intestinal debility.
Prepared as	Infusion, tincture

Angelica
ANGELICA ARCHANGELICA

Also known as	Archangelica officinalis
Where found	Europe and Asia
Appearance	A herbaceous plant growing up to two metres high.
Part used	Roots, seeds and leaves

Therapeutic uses	Angelica is a stimulating expectorant usually combined with other remedies in the treatment of bronchial affections, including dry coughs, bronchial catarrh, asthma, chronic bronchitis and feverish colds. It is also helpful in rheumatic complaints and to increase the menstrual flow. The seeds are considered to be the most active part, although all parts of the plant are similar in action. An infusion can be made from one ounce of the bruised root to one pint of boiling water. The dose is one or two tablespoonfuls two or three times a day. This remedy is contraindicated in diabetes and pregnancy.
Prepared as	Infusion, decoction, tincture

Aniseed
PIMPINELLA ANISUM

Also known as	Anise
Where found	Grown in Southern Europe, North Africa, India and South America
Appearance	White flowering garden herb with feathery leaves, growing to about 50cm high.
Part used	Seeds

Therapeutic uses	A valuable bronchial remedy, indicated in dry coughs to aid expectoration. One teaspoonful of the bruised seeds is infused in five fluid ounces of boiling water, strained and cooled and given in doses of one teaspoonful. Oil of aniseed has been used in herbal preparations for both asthma and bronchitis. Aniseed also helps relieve flatulence and colic.
Prepared as	Powder, infusion, tincture

Asafoetida
FERULA FOETIDA

Also known as	Food of the Gods
Where found	Iran and Afghanistan
Appearance	A plant growing to two metres or more, producing yellow-green flowers and reddish-brown fruits.
Part used	Resin from the root
Therapeutic uses	Asafoetida has been in use for centuries. It is an antispasmodic and expectorant used in bronchitis, asthma and whooping cough, but because of its strong offensive garlic-like odour it is mainly supplied for the manufacture of pills and tablets. It is, however, used in curry sauces. Asafoetida is also antiflatulent and

nervine. One herbal tablet manufacturer combines asafoetida with hops, scullcap, valerian and gentian. It has also been combined with juniper and capsicum as a treatment for back and kidney problems. Unfortunately, asafoetida has had a reputation for being one of the more adulterated remedies.

Prepared as	Tablets

Bayberry
MYRICA CERIFERA

Also known as	Candle Berry
Where found	United States
Appearance	Shrub up to 8ft high with shiny leaves and globular berries
Part used	Bark
Therapeutic uses	A valuable tonic and cleanser for the whole system. It improves circulation and removes catarrh from the stomach.
Prepared as	Powder, fluid extract, tincture, decoction.

Black Cohosh
CIMICIFUGA RACEMOSA

Also known as	Squaw Root
Where found	United States and Canada

Appearance	A tall herbaceous plant with white feathery flowers
Part used	Rhizome
Therapeutic uses	A general blood purifier and nervine tonic, with antispasmodic, anti-flatulent and sedative properties. It has been used in whooping cough. Small doses only are prescribed as in large doses it may cause nausea and vomiting.
Prepared as	Infusion, decoction, syrup, tincture

Boneset
EUPATORIUM PERFOLIATUM

Also known as	Feverwort
Where found	A common meadow plant in Europe and the United States
Appearance	A perennial growing to about a metre in height with hairy stems. It produces an abundance of white flowers.
Part used	Herb
Therapeutic uses	The warm infusion produces perspiration and is used in colds, bronchial catarrh, flu and fevers. Large doses are emetic and purgative. It is best combined with other remedies, such as elderflowers and catnep.
Prepared as	Infusion and tincture

Cardamom
ELETTARIA CARDAMOMUM

Also known as	Malabar Cardamom
Where found	Ceylon and India
Appearance	Forest plant with large smooth, dark green leaves and small yellowish flowers
Parts used	Fruits, seeds and oil
Therapeutic uses	An aromatic herb mainly used in the treatment of flatulence and to improve digestion.
Prepared as	Powder, liquid extract, tincture

Catnep
NEPETA CATARIA

Also known as	Catmint
Where found	Europe. A common British garden plant.
Appearance	A member of the nettle family, it grows about 30cm high. The leaves and stems are covered in fine hairs.
Part used	Herb
Therapeutic uses	The infusion produces perspiration and is useful in colds, flu and fevers. It will also help to settle the stomach when there is excess wind. For asthma and bronchitis it is combined with equal parts of elderflowers and boneset.
Prepared as	Infusion, tincture

Chamomile, Wild
MATRICARIA CHAMOMILLA

Also known as	German Chamomile
Where found	Corn fields in Europe
Appearance	Herb with small cushion-like flowers in profusion
Part used	Flowers
Therapeutic uses	A popular herbal "tea", which has anti-inflammatory and antispasmodic properties. It is also a valuable gastro-intestinal tonic and stimulating nervine. Its main action seems to be on the nervous system. It reduces flatulence and abdominal distension and eases colicky pains and spasms in the colon.
Prepared as	Infusion, tincture

Chamomile, Common
ANTHEMIS NOBILIS

Also known as	Belgian Chamomile
Where found	A favourite garden herb, it grows abundantly in France and Belgium, and is also widely cultivated.
Appearance	A herb resembling a large daisy with white flowers and yellow centres

Part used	Flowers and herb
Therapeutic uses	An antispasmodic indicated in stomach and intestinal disorders. Very useful in heartburn, simple indigestion, flatulence, colic and debilitated states of the colon – conditions which can aggravate asthma attacks. It is widely prescribed for nervous and hysterical conditions.
Prepared as	Infusion (chamomile tea), fluid extract, tincture

Chickweed
STELLARIA MEDIA

Also known as	Starweed
Where found	A common plant in England
Appearance	A small plant, usually regarded as a weed, which produces small white flowers continually through the summer months.
Part used	Herb
Therapeutic uses	A demulcent used in the treatment of irritable skin diseases, and for inflammatory and irritating conditions of the lungs, including asthma and bronchitis. Its use for both skin and lung is interesting as many people with eczema, for example, also suffer with asthma. The

epithelium of the skin is similar to that in the lung. Chickweed is used both internally and externally. An infusion can be used as a soothing lotion, or the herb can be made into an ointment.

Prepared as   Infusion, decoction, tincture, ointment

Cinnamon
CINNAMOMUM ZEYLANICUM

Where found	A native plant of Ceylon
Appearance	A tree growing up to 30ft.
Part used	Bark
Therapeutic uses	A pleasantly aromatic herb with carminative, antiseptic and astringent properties. An effective remedy for vomiting and nausea, and will give relief in flatulence and diarrhoea.
Prepared as	Oil, medicinal water, tincture, powder

Cramp Bark
VIBURNUM OPULUS

Also known as	Snowball Tree, Guelder Rose
Where found	Europe and the United States

Appearance	Strong-growing bush with white ball-shaped flowers
Part used	Bark
Therapeutic uses	Cramp bark, as its name suggests, is an antispasmodic. It is also an excellent nervine. It has been successfully used in combination with other nervines and anti-spasmodics for asthma and nervous hysteria.
Prepared as	Decoction and tincture

Echinacea
ECHINACEA ANGUSTIFOLIA

Also known as	Cone Flower
Where found	American prairies
Appearance	Herb of medium height
Part used	Rhizome
Therapeutic uses	A natural antibiotic, antiseptic and alterative. Helps to clear the blood of toxic material. Improves appetite and digestion.
Prepared as	Decoction and tincture

Elecampane
INULA HELENIUM

Also known as	Wild Sunflower
Where found	Widely distributed throughout Europe and Asia

Appearance	A large herbaceous plant with yellow flowers
Part used	Root
Therapeutic uses	An expectorant and antiseptic, which helps to clear mucus from the chest. It is used in coughs, catarrh, bronchial asthma and other respiratory diseases. According to Culpeper it "helps the cough, shortness of breath and wheezing in the lungs". It works better in combination with Horehound and Thyme.
Prepared as	Decoction, tincture

Garlic
ALLIUM SATIVUM

Where found	Universally cultivated
Appearance	Similar to a shallot
Part used	Bulb
Therapeutic uses	An expectorant and natural antibiotic, ideal for those with asthma, breathing difficulties, coughs and catarrh. It will cleanse the lungs and expel mucus. May be taken in tablet or capsule form, or a syrup can be made with garlic juice and honey in equal parts, or by using one part fresh root to two parts boiling water, allowing to steep for

several hours and then adding honey. Garlic also reduces the level of cholesterol in the blood.

Prepared as   Oil (in capsules), juice, tablets and tincture

Gentian
GENTIANA LUTEA

Also known as	Yellow Gentian
Where found	Alpine plant in Europe
Appearance	A hardy herbaceous perennial bearing clusters of large orange-yellow flowers.
Part used	Root
Therapeutic uses	One of the finest herbal tonics. It is very bitter to the taste even when greatly diluted, but it boosts appetite and aids digestion. Gentian is often prescribed when there is a general debility. It is better to combine small doses of the medicine with an aromatic herb such as Cardamoms to help camouflage the bitter taste.
Prepared as	Tincture and powder (use a quarter of a teaspoonful infused in a cupful of boiling water and sweetened with honey).

Goldenseal
HYDRASTIS CANADENSIS

Also known as   Yellow Root

Where found   Cultivated in North America

Appearance   Tall-growing herb with disagreeable odour

Part used   Rhizome

Therapeutic uses   A most important herb in herbal medicine. It is an anti-inflammatory which is particularly soothing to the epithelium – the skin surface both outside and inside the body, which serves as a protective covering. Epithelial cells line not only the respiratory tract, but also the digestive and urinary tracts. In these situations the lining secretes mucus and is known as a mucous membrane. Hydrastis is a remedy, therefore, for catarrhal as well as inflammatory disorders affecting the mouth, throat, stomach, intestinal lining and lungs. It is also antiseptic, antifungal and laxative, as well as being a blood purifier. Another use is in eye lotions and for inflammatory skin diseases. Goldenseal is one of the more expensive herbs, but it is used only in small doses, usually in combination with other

remedies. Large doses are toxic. It
is contraindicated in pregnancy.
Recommended to be taken under
the supervision of a qualified
herbalist.

Prepared as   Decoction, powder, tincture

Hops
HUMULUS LUPULUS

Where found	Cultivated in most parts of the world
Appearance	A climbing vine
Part used	Strobiles
Therapeutic uses	A nervine tonic and sedative mainly used in combination with other remedies for indigestion and as a liver and gall bladder remedy. It allays pain and promotes restful sleep. May be used in combination with other remedies in nervous asthma.
Prepared as	Tincture, infusion

Lady's Slipper
CYPRIPEDIUM PUBESCENS

Also known as	Nerve Root
Where found	Europe and the United States
Appearance	A delicate wild orchid at present in short supply, and, therefore, highly expensive. Attempts to

grow it commercially for medicinal use have not been very successful.

Part used   Rhizome

Therapeutic uses   A most effective nervine used to allay disorders of a nervous origin, including emotional tension. It helps to induce natural sleep. It is also antispasmodic and relaxing.

Prepared as   Powder, decoction, fluid extract and tincture

Lemon Balm
MELISSA OFFICINALIS

Also known as   Sweet Balm

Where found   Southern Europe, but is now a common garden herb in Britain.

Appearance   It belongs to the nettle family to which it bears some resemblance, but has a strong lemon smell.

Parts used   Leaves, whole herb

Therapeutic uses   Carminative. A useful and safe remedy for the stomach. It relieves flatulence and gastric upsets. It has antifungal properties and is also indicated in fevers. It will induce sweating. An infusion of the leaves (one ounce to one pint of boiling water) can be drunk as required.

Marshmallow
ALTHAEA OFFICINALIS

Also known as	Schloss tea
Where found	Throughout Europe
Appearance	A strong-growing herb which is usually found in watery places
Parts used	Leaves and root
Therapeutic uses	An emollient, demulcent and anti-inflammatory, soothing to both the respiratory tract and the stomach. A useful herb in bronchial troubles. The infusion is soothing to the throat and chest. It is often combined with Slippery Elm and Chickweed.
Prepared as	Infusion (of leaves), decoction (of root), syrup and tincture

Nettle
URTICA DIOICA

Also known as	Stinging Nettles
Where found	Nettles grow on waste ground and near hedges.
Appearance	A perennial growing to about 120 centimetres high with prickly hairs.
Parts used	Leaves, seeds or whole herb
Therapeutic uses	The main action is on the kidneys, but nettles are also used

in skin and lung diseases. The plant is rich in vitamins and minerals and makes an excellent blood tonic for anaemic conditions. A syrup made from the roots or leaves was recommended by Culpeper as a remedy for wheezing and shortness of breath – "a sure medicine to open the passages of the lungs". He also noted that "it helps to expectorate phlegm".

Prepared as   Infusion, tincture

Poplar
POPULUS TREMULOIDES

Also known as	Quaking Aspen
Where found	North America and Europe
Appearance	A large tree
Part used	Bark
Therapeutic uses	A good general tonic: improves appetite and digestion. A useful medicine to take during convalescence. Poplar has also been found to be beneficial in cases of muscular rheumatism and arthritis.
Prepared as	Decoction, powder and tincture

Prickly Ash
XANTHOXYLUM AMERICANUM

Also known as	Toothache Tree
Where found	Canada and the United States
Appearance	Medium-sized tree
Parts used	Bark and berries
Therapeutic uses	The berries have both stimulant and antispasmodic properties. Also helpful as a circulatory tonic and in treatment for chronic rheumatism
Prepared as	Decoction, fluid extract and tincture

Pulsatilla
ANEMONE PULSATILLA

Also known as	Wind Flower
Where found	Britain and Europe
Part used	Leaves
Therapeutic uses	Sedative, nervine and antispasmodic. Used only in small doses – usually in combination with other remedies – for stress conditions. It is beneficial to mucous membranes and helps alleviate catarrh.
Prepared as	Infusion and tincture. Only used in small doses.

Red Sage
SALVIA OFFICINALIS

Also known as	Garden Sage
Where found	Commonly cultivated as a culinary herb in Europe and the United States.
Appearance	A herb growing to about 12cm with purplish flowers.
Part used	Leaves
Therapeutic uses	It is an astringent with stimulating and carminative properties. Useful in debilitated conditions. The infusion is used as a gargle in sore throat and laryngitis. Helps prevent excessive perspiration.
Prepared as	Infusion and tincture. Not to be taken in pregnancy.

Stone Root
COLLINSONIA CANADENSIS

Also known as	Heal-all
Where found	Canada
Appearance	Woodland plant with large greenish-yellow flowers.
Part used	Root
Therapeutic uses	Gastrointestinal tonic, antispasmodic and urinary agent. Has a reputation for clearing stones from the bladder.
Prepared as	Decoction and tincture

Thyme
THYMUS VULGARIS

Where found	Common garden plant
Appearance	Small perennial herb, tiny leaves
Part used	Herb
Therapeutic uses	Antispasmodic and tonic. Contains thymol, a strong antiseptic, useful in irritable coughs and catarrh. Culpeper observed that "it purges the body of phlegm and is excellent for shortness of breath".
Prepared as	Infusion, sweetened with honey and given in tablespoonful doses.

Valerian
VALERIAN OFFICINALIS

Also known as	All Heal
Where found	Near streams, rivers and ditches in Britain
Appearance	Grows to about a metre in height with pinkish white flowers.
Part used	Rhizome
Therapeutic uses	Nervine, sedative and antispasmodic. Excellent for relieving nervous tension and debility. A remedy for asthma induced by stress.
Prepared as	Decoction, fluid extract and tincture

Vervain
VERBENA OFFICINALIS

Also known as	Herb of Grace
Where found	By roadsides and in meadows in Britain
Appearance	A perennial trailing herb bearing small pale-lilac flowers.
Part used	Leaves
Therapeutic uses	A nervine tonic, which also improves liver function and clears mucus from the body. Culpeper recommended it for "coughs, wheezings and shortness of breath". In the first stage of fevers and colds it produces perspiration and helps to reduce temperature. Its nervine properties lift depression and ease tension. Vervain is emetic in large doses. Best used in combination with Horehound.
Prepared as	Infusion and tincture

Wild Yam
DIOSCOREA VILLOSA

Also known as	Colic Root
Where found	Tropical countries, United States and Canada
Appearance	A perennial climbing plant.

Part used	Root
Therapeutic uses	Used in asthma for its antispasmodic properties. In small doses it will relieve nausea, flatulence and colic. Also prescribed for cramping pains, painful periods, uterine pain and rheumatism. Large doses are emetic.
Prepared as	Decoction, fluid extract and tincture. Note: dried root quickly loses its therapeutic potency.

Wood Betony
BETONICA OFFICINALIS

Also known as	Bishopswort
Where found	Woodland in Europe
Appearance	A broad-leaved plant with spikes of red flowers spotted with white.
Parts used	Leaves or whole herb
Therapeutic uses	A general tonic particularly useful in conditions where both nerves and stomach are involved, such as stomach pain and headache due to digestive upset. Helps alleviate dyspepsia.
Prepared as	Decoction, infusion and tincture

Yarrow

ACHILLEA MILLEFOLIUM

Also known as	Nosebleed, Milfoil, Thousand-leaf
Where found	Roadsides, meadows and wasteground in Britain
Appearance	An upright plant growing to about 61 cm with leaves divided into a multitude of parts, hence the name thousand-leaf. The flowers are white or pink with yellowish centres.
Part used	Herb
Therapeutic uses	The hot infusion induces sweating making it an excellent remedy in colds, flu and bronchial catarrh: combine with peppermint.
Prepared as	Infusion, tincture

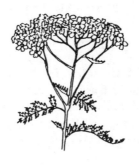

Yarrow

Chapter 25

Professional Advice

This book is aimed at giving those with asthma and related respiratory problems basic information and guidance on the herbal and naturopathic approaches to treatment. Much quicker results, however, can often be achieved by consulting a fully qualified herbal or naturopathic practitioner.

Naturopaths trained at the British College of Naturopathy and Osteopathy in London and admitted to the Register of Naturopaths have the letters ND MRN after their names.

They are specialists in the non-drug treatment of a wide variety of conditions, including asthma, although many naturopaths are also qualified osteopaths and tend to specialise in musculoskeletal problems.

The National Institute of Medical Herbalists, founded in 1864, is the oldest established body of practising medical herbalists in the world. Members can be found in most towns in the UK. The easiest way to find out if there is one near you is to look under 'Herbalists' in Yellow Pages, Thomson's, or other local directory.

The aim of both naturopathy and herbal medicine is not just to relieve symptoms but to offer the sufferer an increased level of general health and wellbeing.

Glossary of Common Medical Terms

Very often when reading, or on having a medical consultation, words are used which may not be familiar. This list will help to make some of the more common ones a little clearer.

Abortifacient
A drug or other substance which produces abortion.

Acholia
A deficiency of bile secretion.

Acidosis
A condition in which the blood becomes more acid. Symptoms include vomiting and drowsiness.

Acrophobia
Fear of heights.

Adhesion
The sticking together of two surfaces in the body that should be separate. Adhesions may be a complication of surgery, but often are the result of inflammation. Bowel adhesions are common and can lead to intestinal obstruction.

Affinity
Usually refers to the attraction of two substances. In herbal medicine the term is used to denote that a remedy has an inherent means of finding its way

to a specific tissue. It is of interest that the active principles of Convallaria, for example, find their way to the heart where they act therapeutically.

Alterative A medicine that beneficially alters the process of nutrition and restores the normal function of an organ or bodily system. In herbal medicine it usually refers to a remedy that purifies the blood by improving the function of the organs, such as liver and kidneys, which are involved in this process.

Amenorrhoea Absence of menstrual periods during the years when they should normally be present.

Analgesic A medicine that blocks or relieves pain.

Anodyne A medicine that alleviates pain – physical or mental.

Anthelmintic A medicine that is used to rid the body of intestinal worms.

Antiphlogistic A medicine, or agent, which reduces inflammation or fever.

Antipyretic A medicine, or method, used to lower the body temperature to normal. In naturopathic medicine, cold baths, and spongeing or application of ice packs are used to combat fever.

Antiseptic A medicine, or other substance, that prevents putrefaction.

Antispasmodic   A remedy that prevents or relieves colic or spasms. Among the most potent antispasmodics derived from plants are belladonna and opium. Naturopathic antispasm is achieved with the application of hot compresses and fomentations.

Aperient   A remedy that produces a natural movement of the bowels.

Aphrodisiac   A substance that is reputed to produce sexual desire and stimulate the sexual organs.

Ascorbic acid   The chemical name for Vitamin C.

Astringent   Binding or contracting tissues.

Cardiac   Relating to the heart, either a medicine, or disease, that alters heart function.

Carminative   A medicine that eases griping pains and flatulence in the bowel.

Cathartic   A strong laxative, or purgative, producing evacuation of the bowels.

Climacteric   The whole transition period during which a woman's fertility declines and ceases and other bodily changes take place which lead to senescence.

Corrective   Correcting or counteracting the harmful and restoring to a healthy state.

Debility   Feebleness of health; run down.

Degenerative   A disease that results in destruction or disintegration of tissue.

Demulcent	A soothing medicine, mostly applied to those that act on the gastrointestinal canal.
Deobstruent	Removing obstructions and opening the ducts and other natural passages of the body.
Diaphoretic	A substance that induces perspiration.
Diuretic	A substance that increases the flow of urine.
Dysmenorrhoea	Excessive pain during menstruation
Dyspnoea	Breathlessness
Emetic	Any substance that causes vomiting.
Emmenagogue	A remedy that brings on the menstrual period.
Emollient	A medicine that softens, soothes and lubricates skin and internal tissues.
Geriatrics	The branch of medicine that specialises in diseases and care of the elderly.
Glycosuria	An excess of sugar in the urine.
Haematemesis	Vomiting of blood
Haematology	The study of diseases of the blood.
Haemoptysis	Coughing up of blood
Haemostatic	A substance that checks bleeding and aids clotting of the blood.
Insecticide	Any substance fatal to insects.
Laxative	A substance that induces gentle, and easy bowel movement.
Leucorrhoea	A mucous discharge from the

female genital organs, previously known as "the whites".

Maceration The process by which the medicinal properties of herbs are extracted and made into liquid extracts.

Menorrhagia Excessive flow of menstrual blood.

Menopause The final menstrual period.

Metrorrhagia Irregular bleeding from the uterus not associated with menstruation.

Myalgia Muscular pain; muscular rheumatism.

Narcotic A drug that produces drowsiness, sleep, stupor and insensibility.

Nephritic Relating to the kidneys.

Nervine A remedy that relieves a nerve disorder and restores the nervous system to its normal state.

Oxytocic A drug that causes contractions of the uterus and hastens childbirth.

Parturient A remedy used during childbirth.

Purgative A medicine taken to evacuate the bowels, but one that is much stronger than a laxative or aperient.

Resolvent A drug, application, or other substance that reduces swellings and tumours.

Rubefacient A treatment that produces redness, inflammation and blisters of the skin; a counter-irritant (rubefy = make red).

Sedative A remedy soothing to the nervous system; a tranquilliser.

Soporific	Promoting sleep.
Stimulant	A remedy that produces a rapid increase in vital energy of part or of the whole body.
Stomachic	Relating to the stomach; a remedy that aids the normal function of the stomach, promoting proper digestion and appetite.
Stricture	The narrowing of any of the natural passages of the body, such as the urethra, the bowel or the gullet.
Styptic	A substance that checks bleeding.
Sudorific	A remedy that produces heavy perspiration.
Tonic	A medicine that invigorates or tones up a part or the whole of the body and promotes wellbeing.
Urology	The branch of medicine that deals with diseases affecting the urinary tract.
Urticaria	A disease allied to asthma and hay fever, but affecting the skin which erupts into irritating wheals.
Vermifuge	A medicine that expels worms from the body.
Vulnerary	An ointment or treatment that promotes the healing of wounds.